Copyright Judith Cutler, 2023

Made in the USA

Author Judith Cutler

Illustrator, Editor, Publisher Jess Perna

Visit and Comment on our Blog

vaginalprolapse.blogspot.com

```
I0104161
```

This book is dedicated to

Dr. Martina Chiodi

Las Brisas OB/GYN

Murrieta, CA

For giving me back my freedom.

Thank you, love and gratitude to Edith founder of the Facebook group:

Colpocleisis, Surgical Vaginal Closing, Colpectomy, LeFort

and the incredibly supportive women in the group.

I strongly suggest joining the group for the help and support you need. It is private and confidential.

Pre-teen us: *"What is going to come out of where every month?!!!"*

"Yes! But, only for about 40 years."

"What is going to go in where? Really to make a baby!"

"What??? The baby is going to come out of where???"

So, thousands of diaper changes later, thousands of dirty dishes, thousands of meals prepared and millions of days of house cleaning and then the whole structure collapses and we are left trying to figure out what to do about it. No one told us this part. Sooo along comes Edith and Facebook to the rescue! What did our mothers, grandmothers, great-grandmothers do? No FB.

Thank you to my wonderful son Jess who illustrated and designed the cover, proofread, edited and published the book with patience and care. He took care of me every step of the way as he always does.

Thank you to my son Mark for keeping me entertained with conversation and stories as he always does.

Mark's rescue cats Maggie and Oliver kept me entertained through photos and videos of their antics.

You can recover more cheerfully watching cat videos. I promise!

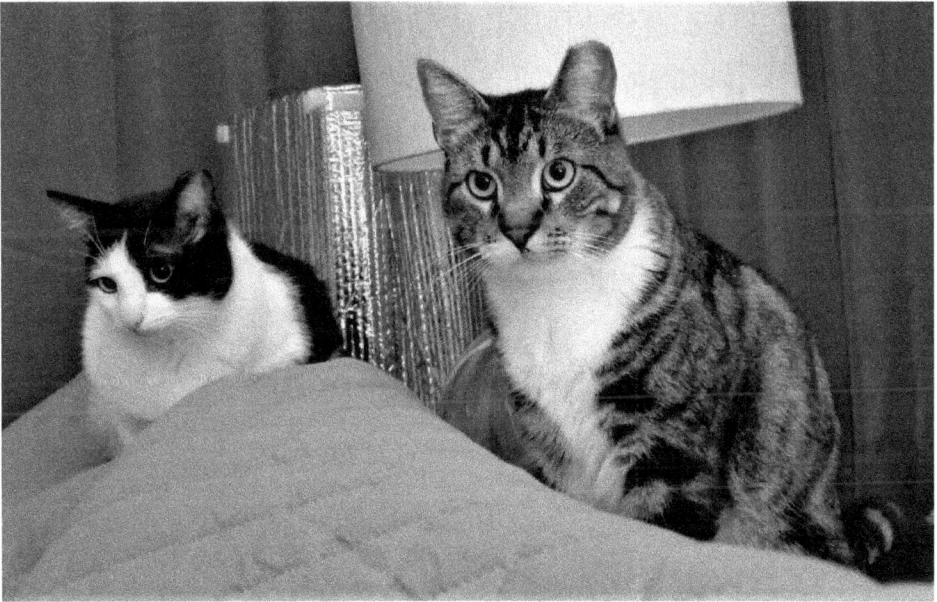

Maggie & Oliver Perna

The Cave In

After two years of complete vaginal prolapse (Stage 4), I decided to take a close-up look at the monster that was ruining and running my life. Up until then I had seen it from a distance in the bathroom mirror. It appeared to be the size of a tennis ball. I put one foot on the bathtub ledge and aimed a large hand mirror upward. Due to the prolapse, tissue that was previously hidden from view could now be seen on the outside including the approximately 3-inch incision scar from my hysterectomy done over 20 years before. The scar was beige, except for a white spot on the end. Hmmm, what's that? It concerned me.

I looked up some possibilities online, learning that 90% of the time a similar spot is nothing serious. The other 10% of the time it could be a pre-cancer of the cervix. I did not have a cervix anymore, but I had what was referred to as a cervical rim.

When I had my hysterectomy, the surgeon said I never needed to be examined by a gynecologist again since there was nothing left to examine. He said I was free from worry since I no longer had ovaries. I simply had what was referred to as a vaginal vault. Basically, a passage ending at the back wall.

If my vaginal vault had not prolapsed, I would not have seen the white spot. It needed to be checked and I knew I would not rest easy until it was confirmed by a physician not to be a threat.

My HMO plan necessitates a referral from my GP before I can consult a specialist. I promptly made an appointment and hoped the GP could just do a Pap Smear on the cervical rim and be done with it. However, the GP said it needed a needle biopsy, for which I would have to see a gynecologist. The first gynecologist I was referred to had just recently stopped taking my insurance plan. The second one, Dr. Martina Chiodi in Murrieta, California agreed to see me right away since there was a concern.

Even though I knew she had seen this kind of problem before I was embarrassed and nervous. It isn't easy to present something so unsightly even to a doctor. She was extremely kind and gave the gentlest exam I ever experienced by a gynecologist. She did a totally painless needle biopsy. I actually did not know she had started when she declared herself finished!

She said, "This prolapse has to be fixed. Otherwise, it will get lesions and then you will have a big problem. You cannot leave this outside your body!" I asked what she recommended. She said there is a repair surgery and she could recommend someone since she doesn't do it. I told her I read about that surgery and felt it was a catastrophic failure since 50% of the time it has to be redone and can still fail. I also was not willing to risk the side effects I read about in science articles.

"Is there a plan B," I asked?

"There is," she said, "It's called a LeFort Colpocleisis. I do them all the time. But you are still young and if you have this surgery, you can NEVER have intercourse again. It closes off the vaginal opening making it only 1 inch deep and much narrower." (Total Colpocleisis is another type of this surgery. I cannot advise which is best for you. It is for you to look into and decide.)

"Sounds like the best option." I replied. I told her I read about that surgery on a doctor's blog, but did not know the name of it. She said it has a 95% success rating by patients. I mentioned the article I read was by a physician who said closing off the vagina is sometimes the only option. He said sometimes it in can result in incontinence. I asked her if that was a risk. She said it only happened to one of her patients. She discovered the way to tell if it was a risk was if you lost urine when you pushed upward on the prolapse. I said that did not happen to me. I had to push the prolapse back away from the urethra to be able to pee. She called it "splinting."

12 years prior I lost interest in having sex with men, so intercourse no longer mattered. "Let's do the surgery!" I am 75 years old and my first consideration was comfort.

She agreed it was the best option for me and said she performed the surgery at a surgical center nearby her office. Her schedule was not overbooked and I could have it done in 2 weeks. I scheduled the procedure before leaving her office. I was given a prescription for the surgery to take to my GP for insurance approval. My son drove me straight to the GP and within a few hours I had the written approval that my insurance would cover all costs. I had an HMO and Medicare.

The next step was to get an EKG at the GP's office 5 days later. An EKG was necessary to be to be cleared for surgery to determine if it was safe for me to go under anesthesia. At that appointment is when things started to get complicated. The EKG showed something called a Left Branch Bundle Block in my heart. The GP said I had to get clearance for surgery from a cardiologist and gave me a referral. The cardiologist was booked for a month but after the GP's office called in a favor, they agreed to see me immediately!

By immediately, I mean I received a call telling me to get to the cardiologist within 30 minutes for an exam. I had 5 minutes to jump in the shower and dress for the 20-minute drive to his office. The GPS sent us in circles and we were a few minutes late. It didn't make a difference since we had to wait for an hour to see the doctor. I was a nervous wreck by then. If he did not approve the surgery, I didn't know what I would do.

The gynecologist said I had to have the surgery or be in danger of lesions. If the cardiologist wouldn't approve me for surgery the only option was a local anesthetic, but the surgical center doesn't administer those. Dr. Chiodi was the only one in the area doing the surgery.

I was so nervous I knew my blood pressure would be high. The cardiologist's office was cold, and I cold rooms can elevate your blood pressure. Sure enough, it was up 30 points compared to a few days before when taken at my GP's office. I thought he would turn me down based on that, but he didn't even mention it.

What he wanted to know was how I felt. He could see my leg muscles were developed so I was telling the truth about how active I am. He said as long as I had no symptoms and felt strong, he would approve the surgery. There was no physical exam. No treadmill, just a discussion. He asked my son if he could vouch for me as to my physical fitness and exercise routine. My son told him that when we take walks together, he often has trouble keeping up with me!

The doctor told me to come back in 3 months for a follow up, and approved the surgery. I was relieved and stunned! Grateful beyond words, I went home and called my other son and friends with the good news.

There was still one little dark cloud hovering over me that kept me in its shadow for the next few days…my Left Branch Bundle Block. The cardiologist said even though he approved my surgery, some anesthesiologists would not treat someone with that heart condition unless they had the results of a nuclear stress test first. He couldn't guarantee I'd be approved to get my surgery when I'm at the surgery center.

Everyone was reassuring me, including the scheduler at the gynecologist's office, but I needed this to happen so badly that I wasn't going to feel any comfort until the procedure was underway.

Getting a blood test for the gynecologist was another ordeal. The directions for the lab took us to the wrong building. We had an appointment, but sat in a waiting room for half an hour while others who came in after us were taken first. There was no receptionist. Finally, when one of the technicians came out to call someone else, I asked why we were still not called. She looked at my form said, "That's because you're scheduled at the lab in the next building."

There was no sign on the door indicating there were two labs with the exact same name! We hurried next door and found the correct lab. I asked the lab tech why there wasn't a sign on the door mentioning the other lab. She said, "Oh, yes that happens all the time!" That was it. No 'sorry'. No, 'you are right, we should have a sign'. She just laughed.

My son said while he was waiting for me an elderly couple discovered they were supposed to be in the building we just came from. One had a walker. I guess watching needy patients scurry between the two buildings is a source of entertainment for the lab techs.

The reason I mention these random, annoying problems is because more often than not, these are the sorts of things that happen when going through the healthcare system. I hope you get lucky and all goes smoothly, however if it doesn't, don't feel alone. Plow through until you get the help you need!

Five days before the surgery one of the last things I had to do was go back to the gynecologist with my cardiologist approval form to get final pre-op instructions. It was the usual advice like not to eat for 12 hours prior to surgery. I signed the agreements stating I understood the risks of surgery and once again addressed the fact that yes, I knew I would never again be able to have intercourse. They want to make sure they aren't sued later because the patient was surprised at this extreme limitation. I don't blame them.

As always, the prolapse hurt, my activities were a strain but knowing it would soon be gone made life so much easier.

The next few days were filled with getting the apartment ready; cleaning, changing sheets, buying supplies, etc.

Later in this book will be a list of how I prepared my home and what I used to recover after the operation. You can tear the page out to take to the store. After all you won't need the list twice! If you are reading an electronic copy of the book, just take your device to the store.

4 Days Until Surgery

Following in the footsteps of General Dwight D. Eisenhower, I plotted my pre and post operation as carefully as he planned the Normandy invasion. Well, maybe mine was a little less complex, but I believe in planning for a great outcome. For one, it keeps our minds focused on the goal and helps keep the jitters to a minimum.

The first thing I did was to join a wonderful Facebook group of supportive women who had been through the surgery and some who were waiting their turns. The women were all generous with their time and advice. The group is called "Colpocleisis, Surgical Vaginal Closing, Colpectomy, LeFort." It is a private group open only to women over 50 years of age. For admittance they must answer a few questions to be part of the group. It was started in 2021 by a woman who at first did not give her whole name and later on did. I joined under an assumed name since I was embarrassed to have anyone know about my condition. This is often the case when people communicate online about such personal subjects. I noticed some of the names listed a hobby rather than an individual's identity.

After being in the group for a few weeks, going through the surgery and recovering I realized there was no shame necessary. I was proud to be a member of such a group of caring, kind and courageous women. However, by that time I couldn't figure out how to change my name on Facebook.

Eventually I left the group and rejoined under my real name.

Hearing recovery stories of other women with this condition provided me strength, a road map to follow and I felt less alone. Rarely someone wrote the surgery was not a success for them. I actually only saw one such post. Most of the women were raving about how well they felt and that the surgery had given their life back! The women also shared the supplies they used, doctors they engaged and details of their lives. They even told of their continued sex lives *without* intercourse, something referred to as outercourse. For anyone facing the possibility of Colpocleisis surgery I strongly recommend joining the group. The group has a valuable, hard to come by, directory of recommended surgeons and their locations.

My goal for this book is to give you strength, encouragement and empower you with information about a condition that is not talked about enough. It is extremely important to have easily accessible support and to get your questions answered. I can only tell my story. While there are many things you and I will have in common, the women in the group may have a situation more similar to yours.

The doctors do not give you a playbook for every bit of your recovery. Their skills lie in the mechanics of surgery and the after care. They haven't had the surgery themselves. They cannot supply emotional support and intimate knowledge which comes from others who have faced this very difficult challenge.

Back to my battle plan:

- A son to drive me to the surgery and fetch me after.
- Checking if I filled out the required medical forms from home. I don't want to sit in the waiting room writing while nervously waiting for my surgery. The surgical center had almost 30 pages of forms. I would never have all the details they wanted memorized.
- Shop for a week's groceries.
- Pre-cook as much as possible so meals can just be heated up.
- Make the bed with several layers of sheets so that remaking the bed is just a matter of pulling the top layers off and a new clean set will be at the ready. I also prepared my easy chair similarly.
- A clean, inexpensive shower curtain liner under the top layer of sheets to

capture any blood seeping through the pads. (As it turned out unnecessary in my case).

- Sanitary pads as bleeding can occur for up to 2 weeks.
- Fiber laxatives and pills of the kind used to prep for a colonoscopy. These to be taken in much smaller doses compared to a colonoscopy prep.
- Unscented baby wipes since toilet paper can be a little too rough for the 4-6 weeks. (Very necessary).
- Witch hazel, aloe gel and Aquaphor to pat on the stitches to facilitate healing and ease itching.
- A handy basket, purse or cloth shopping bag (anything with an arm loop) for carrying around pen, paper, eye glasses, eye glass cleaner, phone, tablet, book, Kindle

and anything else needed to carry around from easy chair to bed. Getting up and down fetching these items won't be easy for the first week. The handy basket means asking others to fetch is kept to a minimum.

- Organize any pain pills or supplements on a tray so they can be brought close by.
- A stack of easy to slip on night clothes and socks.
- Get the house in order: vacuum, clean and then forget about cleaning until I am recovered enough to do it again.
- Pay bills so I don't have to think about them for a few weeks.
- Get some good reading material.
- Set up automatic "out of the office," email reply settings for 48 hours.

- Set up a purse with just ID and insurance cards since I cannot bring money or valuables to the surgery center.
- My 3rd Covid booster was 2 weeks before the surgery. I knew I would not be able to wear a mask during the surgery and wanted the best protection I could have against Covid.
- The day before the surgery I ate a high fiber diet and drank a lot of water. I wanted to be sure to be able to have a bowel movement without struggling as there would be a lot of stitches in the area. I knew I would not be able to bear down.
- By the time I finished all the chores in my battle plan it was time to go get the surgery done. Finally! I was so busy getting ready I did not have

much time to get nervous. I was still waiting to see if at the last minute the anesthesiologist was going to question my EKG and reject my qualification for the procedure. I was so relieved when she just greeted me, gave me a pre-op pain pill and said, "See you inside the OR".

The Surgery Day

My son drove us to the surgery center and kept me company in the waiting room before my operation. We were told to wear masks while waiting which was fine with us. Since Covid-19, we always wear them going to indoor public places.

There was a very low reception desk with no chair for those checking in to sit. I had to stoop over to give them my ID and insurance cards, have the wrist band placed and retrieve my belongings. This arrangement didn't take into account the comfort of those of us waiting for surgery. All of a sudden there was a loud noise and a cackling sound! I jumped! It was the first week of October. Someone had the bright idea to have a Halloween witch electric noise maker screaming at patients and thought that would be welcome. Rattled we sat down to wait.

The waiting area TV station was loudly tuned to the news. Call me picky but having stories of war, mayhem and murder on the screen in a surgery center waiting room is not my idea of stress reduction. It was truly shocking! Every five minutes the witch noise maker would go off. After the third time I complained to the receptionist who said, "Go tell it to the CEO. It was her idea!" To the receptionist's credit she got up and out of her booth to shut it off. I think she was relieved to have a reason to kill that witch.

After 15 minutes the nurse called me into a room to take a rapid Covid test. She swabbed every bit of the inside of both nostrils and told me to put my mask back on. It wasn't pleasant, but it was a good idea since it made me more confident that I would be less likely to catch Covid here. Another nurse came in asking me to sign more forms. Both nurses were very kind, warm and friendly. I had to agree once more I did not care about having intercourse in the future and sign that I understood this surgery is not reversible. She said, "I cannot pronounce the name of your surgery!" I said, "Don't worry, I can't either, but you spelled it correctly!"

After taking my blood pressure they sent me back to await the results of the 15-minute rapid Covid test. The witch had stopped screaming, but the depressing TV news was still blasting away. Fifteen minutes later the nurse summoned me. I said goodbye to my son, sending him home to await the phone call retrieve me. The actual surgery takes 1 hour and a few more hours for prep and recovery. He told me later he had trepidation when he watched the nurse bring me through the doors. When bringing me to past surgeries he never experienced fear before but this time he did. His instincts were good because a problem arose.

As he drove home, he also felt angry and disgusted that medical science had not aggressively perfected the vaginal prolapse surgery. He agreed with my decision to get this procedure and hated the that it was the most logical course. He could not understand why if doctors can repair hearts, reattach limbs, transplant organs, perform brain surgery, etc., why they weren't motivated enough to reliably repair what he called, "the most important body part there is!" That's my boy.

The nurse walked me back to a room that had three curtained beds. The other two beds had patients being prepped. There were a lot of surgery staff performing different duties. I was weighed, escorted to a bed, given a large plastic bag for my belongings and a hospital gown. They weigh patients to determine the correct amount of anesthesia. I changed into the gown in private, then met the anesthesiologist. She was very friendly and said she would be taking care of me and asked if I was allergic to any meds. I told her I was not. Then she offered me acetaminophen. I told her I don't usually take pain meds. She explained I would need less anesthetic with acetaminophen so I agreed to take it. I was given a tiny sip of water for swallowing the pill.

I was asked to lay back on the bed. The nurse on my right put an intravenous needle in a vein on the back of my hand. For some years, the veins in my forearms haven't been very good for IV's so my hand was used. The nurse on my left attached electrodes to my chest and side so they could monitor my heart. They placed long compression stockings on my legs explaining they would prevent blood clots. Next came no-slip socks with treads on the bottoms which I would be wearing home. They covered me with a sheet and a soft warm blanket. I was very comfortable.

Next, they rolled the bed into the OR and asked me to slide on to the operating table. They kept me covered.

They did not put my legs into stirrups until I was asleep for which I was very glad.

My doctor came in, smiled and greeted me. Well, since she was masked her eyes twinkled with a smile. Then they put a soft, plastic mask on my face and said to breathe slowly and I would relax. The next thing I remembered was being woken up in the room where we had started out on this project. A nurse helped me dress. She said I had to wear a urinary catheter home for a week because the doctor had nicked my bladder and it had to rest while it healed. This was an unpleasant shock! I heard there was a rare occurrence of some women wearing a catheter for 2-3 days after the surgery and I had dreaded the idea of it. Now I would have it for a whole week!

The nurse said my bladder would completely heal. They had taken off the compression stockings. I kept on the surgical, non-slip socks they had given me. I was placed in a wheel chair. Outside my son was waiting to take me home.

They helped me into the front seat and the nurse proceeded to give him instructions for the cath bag and my home care. She actually placed the info on the back of the dirty car trunk and stood in the heat telling him in rapid succession how to do something he had no experience with at all. She held up various tubes and components without a visual reference as to how the whole contraption worked together on a human. His requests for further clarification just increased the speed of her instructions and he realized it was futile. The explanations were not done in a caring way and was pretty overwhelming for him.

On the ride home he told me the doctor had called him and told him about the nick in my bladder. She said the prolapse was huge, which made it more difficult to work around. However, she reassured him she had repaired it and I would be totally fine. She said to bring me to her office in a week so she could remove the cath.

He told me about the trepidation he had when he left me that morning and this must have been why. I was just relieved the surgery was over and was not in much pain, although pretty sore. It was similar to the pain of episiotomy stitches after giving birth. I didn't need pain meds then and didn't think I would need them now.

After the anesthetic wore-off, I found I did not need any pain meds and took nothing during the whole recovery period. Pain meds slow digestive transit time making bowel movements much more difficult. I prefer the soreness to that horrific problem. The most pain was going from sitting to standing, standing to sitting or sneezing and coughing.

Once home I was safely tucked into the recliner with the cath bag laying on a towel on the floor as suggested by the nurse. We placed a plastic bag under the towel to protect the carpet from any possible spills. My son and I looked up videos on Youtube about catheter bags to supplement the inadequate instruction from the nurse. For anyone undergoing this surgery it would be advisable to get that info ready in advance for the rare circumstance a catheter is needed.

The worst pain I had was a sore throat. They warned that could happen from intubation. I was asleep when intubated and when extubated. I have no recollection of the procedure, but my throat was extremely sore for 30 hours and then simply stopped hurting and was back to normal.

I had a meal for the first time that day. I kept my legs elevated in the recliner. We kept checking that the urine flow to the bag was continuous. It was easy to move slightly in the wrong position pinning the tube between the sanitary pad, the elastic on my underwear and my thigh muscle. One pinch and the flow would stop which can cause the bladder not to empty. My bladder was supposed to be resting from getting full so the repair of the nick could heal. I checked the flow about every 15 minutes.

The cath bag had to be emptied every 3 hours. I walked slowly to the bathroom holding my son's arm. He was very good about emptying it. I would stand holding on to the bathroom sink as I was still a bit dizzy. The cath bag has a small 3" tube at the bottom that goes into a locked position. To empty it, the person attending it has to wash their hands, then pull it out of the locking sleeve turning it downward toward the toilet and release a valve. The bag then empties. Then the valve must be closed and the small tube secured into locked position again.

I took 3 Dulcolax laxative pills that evening to make sure I would be able to have a bowel movement the next day without tearing the stitches. The perinium is stitched all the way to the anus to make it strong hence the title LeFort, (meaning The Strong in French). This method prevents future prolapses. I also drank a lot of water and herbal tea with honey.

The cath bag has a series of valves and other little gadgets, (I don't have a technical name for them) that allow the tube on the leg to swivel left or right. You lay down and position the swivel toward where the bag is going to be situated. The valves and little gadgets are taped to the leg so that they don't pull on the smaller tube going into the bladder. That tube is held in place by a little balloon in the bladder so it cannot be yanked out.

I had a fitful night of sleep in the easy chair trying to get comfortable. My normal sleeping pattern is to fall asleep on one side and wake up on my stomach. I never remember rolling over. I slept in the chair because I was afraid I would roll over on the cath tube and stop the flow. It was a very uncomfortable night. My son set his clock and woke up every 3 hours to check if the bag needed emptying. It turned out that we could have gotten through at least 6 hours without emptying it even though in the day time 3 hours was the limit. Having had no experience with this we were both nervous about it. We got through the ordeal until morning.

The Recovery Week

Recovery Day 1 - Saturday

The nurse instructed that in order to shower I could just place the catheter bag hook on the towel rack and shower. I was able to stand without dizziness. I managed to dry off and change my clothes, which was a slow process on my own. My son helped with everything else but I was not going to dress in front of him.

I have been very open with my sons about the details of the prolapse and surgery and they were comfortable discussing it with me. However, I did not tell them all the gory details of my condition until it was time to make a decision about whether or not to go through with it. I raised them to be comfortable about the quirks and problems of our bodies. The son I live with was absolutely magnificent about helping with everything I needed. The following week my other son visited and helped with a variety of needed activities. He had volunteered to come from the beginning, but we felt it wasn't necessary.

Here is my method for sitting on the toilet when a cath bag is your constant companion. I hooked the bag onto the drawer handle of the sink cabinet. Then pulled down my underwear and sat, being vigilant to not let the tube get crushed. I lay the bag on the floor on a towel so it would be lower than me, since I couldn't bend over due to the stitches. I used clothes hanger hooks and kitchen tongs to move the cath bag around. This procedure was necessary to be able to poop. Then I reversed the procedure standing up again. The next step was emptying the bag into the toilet. It was a real treat!

The second night I took just one laxative pill. For the rest of the week, I took one pill each morning. I also had the 1 tablespoon of Wheat dextrin fiber powder two times a day mixed in a cup of tea. Once in the morning and at night. Tasteless vegetable fiber dissolves completely in any hot or cold drink. From what I've read Wheat dextrin is gluten free, however for those looking to avoid wheat products a fiber supplement that works very similarly is called Partially Hydrolyzed Guar Gum. Psyllium husk is less ideal as it can be gassy, irritating and create too much of a bulky mass that may increase the recovery discomfort.

I found dressing while sitting on the toilet was the easiest way to begin. First threading the cath bag through one of the underwear leg holes and then following with my leg. Next comes the sanitary pad and struggling to stand up. Bleeding can continue for one to two weeks so keep a batch of pads handy.

The weirdest thing about peeing through the cath tube is feeling the constant urge to pee but having no control. The urine just slowly and continuously flows into the tube. Mentally, I expected to be wetting myself and had to keep remembering the urine was going through the tube. It was very unnerving. I did not adjust to it for the whole week.

All the second day I rested, walked about the apartment a little and rested more while wiggling my ankles at least

5-10 minutes of every hour to help my circulation. By the end of the day, I was bored with sitting and watching TV and reading. I am used to an 80-hour work week running the family business. How many times I had longed for a week off to do nothing and when it actually happened, I wanted to work.

For amusement I spent time every day watching the urine flow in the plastic tube and the bubbles moving up and down the tube. I decide to have some fun with it and name the cath bag "Judy's Dog." It had to be walked to the toilet every few hours.

With the help of my son, I managed to sleep in my bed the second night. It was a carefully planned arrangement involving a lot of pillows at my back so I wouldn't roll over. Then one for between my knees as a I lay on my side with the tube hanging off the bed. The bag placed on a towel with a plastic bag underneath it, checking I hadn't crimped the tube and the flow was continuing. He came in several times during the night to check on me. This arrangement was much better than trying to sleep in the chair. Since my throat wasn't sore any longer, I slept much better the second night.

Recovery Day 2 - Sunday

When you live with the constant pain, discomfort and embarrassment of prolapse there is nothing funny about it. However, with the relief of surgery and an end in sight my sense of humor blossomed out of control.

I posted some of my thoughts in the Facebook group (under my assumed name) and got a lot of laughs. *"The canary died. The Man Cave had a collapse! An "Out of Business" sign was placed in front of the cave."*

Having rested better the night before I felt a little more energetic. I was counting the days until "Judy's Dog" would be sent to live on a *"farm."* I walked around the apartment a little more often and took a second shower. The nurse who told me I could shower with the tube in place failed to mention a crucial bit of information. After two showers the tape holding the bag in place fell off leaving the valves swinging back and forth on my right side and pulling on the tube in my bladder. Extra patches with tape should have been supplied for using a bag for more than a few days. I thought it would stay put since the patch had a notice it had to be removed with alcohol. That was obviously untrue. I had to hold on to the valves to keep them from dragging on my bladder while struggling to dress. Next, I hunted for the perfect tape to secure it again to my thigh.

Having been trained in first aid, I keep an extensive supply of bandages, tape and other equipment. However, these valves were fairly heavy and a lot of tape was needed. The tape pulled on the skin on my thigh when I moved and it hurt. Another irritation was the plastic valves digging into my thigh. I came up with an idea to ease the discomfort. Placing a soft, clean eye glass cleaner cloth between the valves and my skin stopped them from biting into my thigh. Next, I taped the cloth to my skin. Then I taped the valves to the cloth. When I did it incorrectly the thin tube coming out of my body would be crushed and stop the flow. Placing the tape exactly right worked fine. This had to be done every day at least once for the rest of the week. Showering meant doing it all again. The upside was it killed time and brought me closer to the day of getting rid of "Judy's Dog".

Recovery Day 3 - Monday

I had been posting my progress in the Facebook group and writing some of my methods for recovery. Some new members were terrified of the surgery. Those of us who were veterans encouraged and cheered them on. This worked as we could see their attitudes improve and noted how hopeful they all felt.

I was inspired to write this book because as of the time of this writing the only place for emotional support and information about what it's like to go through this procedure is from women on Facebook. What about the multitude of others? Previously, I searched 2 years for information and help. The only thing I found was about the other surgery. There was not one book or blog on the personal experience of someone in my position. All the information was about how to get the repair from a surgery that was far from ideal. I wanted a permanent fix not an iffy repair with a lot of possible adverse side-effects.

I was able to walk around a bit more and kept up with my ankle and arm circulation movements.

Recovery Day 4 – Tuesday

The bleeding had slowed to spotting, although each BM created a certain amount of bleeding. Even without pushing there is still some pressure on the repaired area. I was counting the hours until my appointment on Thursday knowing relief was coming soon.

I realized the cath bag had possibilities no one had thought of before. It should have little floating plastic decorations inside: a fish, a mermaid, a diver, coral reef and tropical undersea plants. As it fills up it would look like a little fish tank! This could entertain countless cath bag users and their friends. I was on to something that could make millions!

My sense of humor kept me going and made friends and family laugh! It was a relief for them not to worry about my mental or physical state.

Recovery Day 5 – Wednesday

There was still some spotting the same as on Tuesday. It was another boring day of rest and feet up. I did not leave the apartment the whole week because of the 26 steps down to the street. Even though they supply a cath leg bag so you can walk outside, the instructions on how to change the valves from the large bag to the smaller leg bag were woefully inadequate. I was afraid of not being capable of securing the different tubes correctly. I watched some videos online, but still did not feel safe to change over to the leg bag. I stayed in the apartment until my doctor appointment on Thursday morning.

I was able to do a little cooking by placing the bag on the kitchen floor and dragging it around. It felt good to be useful.

That night I went to sleep excited at the prospect of having getting rid of "Judy's Dog" but slightly worried the doctor may have a reason to leave it in longer.

Freedom Day – Thursday

I had an early morning appointment and was eager to get going. I placed the bag in a cloth shopping bag and wore a long dress to help hide the tube.

When I walked into the doctor's reception area, I noticed a woman glancing at the tube and quickly looking away. I was past caring about anything embarrassing. It was like going into the delivery of my babies: I just wanted it out! We mother's all know that feeling. It could be in a taxi, a subway platform or Grand Central Station: Deliver already!

Dr. Chiodi was her usual sweet, caring self and said, "Let's get this terrible tube out!" I knew she felt badly about the nick in my bladder and I apologized for my body giving her a hard time.

She explained the longer the prolapse exists the more the skin on it thickens and makes it more difficult to operate on. I had seen graphic videos of the surgery on youtube.com. Part of the surgery is taking the skin off the prolapse, tying up the tissue that is left and tucking it inside the vagina. Then stitches are put in to hold everything together to keep from having another prolapse.

At the time of this writing in November 2022, there is youtube.com instructional video produced by a surgeon showing the surgical technique on a mannequin. It is easier to watch than an actual surgery. If you want a full understanding of the surgical procedure, I highly suggest it. It is entitled "Complete Colpocleisis Model".

youtube.com/watch?v=9sNtCveKAtU

I was glad the skin was removed since my original visit was to make sure there was no cancer forming on the surgical scar from my hysterectomy. Dr. Chiodi explained it was clear since she could not get much of a biopsy. She said that is one way they know it isn't cancer. I was really pleased with that and knowing that scar was removed.

I told her some of the jokes I'd come up with about the situation and she laughed. I was to return in five weeks for a follow up exam.

A fun time was had by all and now I was done with the bag!!! I hope the dog finds a good home somewhere over the rainbow!

The Recovery Adventure Part 2

Now that I could move about more freely, I started talking walks outside. I usually walk 1-3 miles daily. The first day I walked 1 mile and felt really well. I walked just a little slower than usual. It was not a problem to slowly climb the 26 steps back up to my apartment. The next day I was able to walk 2.5 miles at my usual pace of a 20-minute mile. I live in a hilly area so every walk is at least half way uphill. It was encouraging to know I could just continue as always.

The difference in my exercise routine was I could not lift my weights yet or do many stretches. Sitting on the floor touching my toes was not an option. Nor was picking things off the floor. If I dropped something it lay there until I summoned one of my sons to pick it up.

The floors looked like a litter bug lived there! By the end of the second week, I could pick things up from the floor and I felt more normal.

I kept up with light housework since circulation is vital to recovery. After 15 days I was happy to note I had lost 3 lbs. Another perk of the surgery was it lessened my appetite and I was on the road to losing the 25 pounds I had been planning to get rid of for years. Another silver lining!

The most amazing advantage was I could take a long walk and not have to run to the bathroom when I returned. I could wait an hour or so after returning. I even forgot about thinking whether or not I needed to go. For those who don't have urgency problems this development may not seem as exciting as it is to those who have become slaves to it.

I wrote Dr. Chiodi a thank you snail mail letter noting she had given me back my freedom with her tremendous skill and kindness. Thank you isn't enough to convey my gratitude but it will have to do. Since we live in the age of the Google review, I left her a glowing one. I also wrote in the letter that she could show it to anyone who needed the operation and encouragement.

At this point the only discomfort was itching from the stitches which would take about 4 more weeks to be done with their work.

I was so happy I felt like dancing!

Inside Out, Upside Down Vagina

According to everything I have read prolapse happens most often to mothers who have had vaginal deliveries. Most often to those who had a forceps delivery and at least two births. I am one of those mothers.

It may also happen to a young woman who has not had children, however, most often not until after menopause. You can read up on the various ways things can go wrong and how to prevent it from happening at all. There is a variety of advice and opinions.

I have read from many sources that doing Kegel exercises can prevent prolapse. Not in my experience. I have been doing Kegels continuously for 59 years. It keeps me from being incontinent since I can start and stop the urine flow at will. However, it had no impact on prolapse. After having surgery, I can still do strong Kegels. Kegel exercises strengthen the pelvic floor muscles, supporting the uterus, bladder, small intestine and rectum. It is important to do Kegels, also known as pelvic floor muscle training.

I watched a Youtube.com video from a doctor who explained that when vaginal prolapse occurs, the vagina tears away from its supports and turns inside out, literally falling through the vaginal opening. I tried doing Kegels to get the prolapse to come back up into place but since it was no longer connected to the muscles that Kegels use, it was futile.

When I was 51, I had a hysterectomy due to huge fibroids causing bleeding and horrific pain. The surgeon gave me no warning of the possibility of prolapse. I had no idea there even was such a phenomenon. After the hysterectomy, I was on hormone replacement therapy for 15 years. Out of an abundance of caution I stopped after news articles said estrogen could cause breast cancer. Two women I knew with breast cancer also actively discouraged me against continuing HRT. Therefore, a decade ago I discontinued it.

From what I understand now, continuing HRT may have maintained vaginal wall muscle strength and mass that could have prevented prolapse but that is not always the case. There are many women in the prolapse Facebook group who mention they are on hormone replacement therapy. While I may never know if HRT could have prevented the prolapse, I present you this theoretical factor for your health research.

I am now going back on bio-identical hormone replacement because in my case I believe the benefits outweigh the risks. I have had some blood tests including the BRCA test showing that I am not in a high-risk group for breast cancer. Since discontinuing HRT a decade ago, I have lost 2 inches in height and that is not good for my bones.

In my middle sixties I joined a gym and was swimming laps every day. Then I started doing leg press exercises with the machine set to 50 pounds. After a few days I felt a bulge in my vagina that ended right at the entrance. I did some research and found I had a prolapse starting at a stage 2. I read up on it discontinued the leg press. To attempt to reverse the prolapse, I did hundreds of Kegels a day.

I ordered an expensive device from the UK that was supposed to reverse prolapse or at the least keep it from worsening. I faithfully used this battery operated electronic pelvic toner device which had a probe inserted into the vagina and stimulates the muscles to produce powerful Kegel contractions for 45 minutes at a time. It hurt a lot. It delivered small repeating electric shocks. Since it had great reviews, I persevered. After a few years I realized it hadn't made any improvement at all and gave up on it.

At age 73, I suddenly felt my entire vaginal vault drop out in an instant. It was now the size and shape of a tennis ball, very firm and ugly hanging down between my legs. I was unable to pee as it covered the urethra opening. In order to urinate, I had to push it out of the way. I recently learned it is referred to as "splinting".

If the only way to empty your bladder is by splinting that means you are peeing on your hand. It never seemed to be completely empty. After scrubbing my hands, I would dress, leave the bathroom and have to return 5-10 minutes later. Then start the whole terrible process again. This went on 30-40 times a day. Many nights I would wake up at least 12 times and as much as 20. It was exhausting. I never felt I actually had a night's rest for 2 years.

Every time I sat down the bulge would slide back in and it was painful.

That tissue is supposed to be internal and was never meant to be on the outside. The skin on it would get painfully dry making it necessary to put personal lubricant on it each time I used the bathroom. I had to carry some in my purse when I left home.

In order to use a public restroom, I had to carry baby wipes to clean my hands in the toilet stall before going to the communal sink to wash my hands. I did not want to touch anything with my urine-stained hands contaminating the door latch.

The urgency to pee plagued me. Most of the time I had to go through the bathroom routine 4-5 times to go outside for a walk. If I thought my bladder was empty, I would sit down to don my socks and shoes. As soon as I stood, I would have to go again. I would always feel bad, apologizing to those waiting for me.

It became necessary to know the location of every restroom on a route I traveled. If it was by car, I would have to go the minute I stood up. I also had to have extra underwear since the continued application of the lubricant would get messy and damp. Women with prolapse report similar problems.

One of the worst parts is the complete embarrassment that accompanies this problem. My sons were the only people I spoke with about it. I did not tell them the whole extent of the situation, keeping it minimal. I wanted them to know why I stopped going to the gym. I hadn't become lazy, but had a serious issue preventing me from working out with my legs. I walk and dance but they wanted me to do weight training to keep me fit and youthful. I did not describe to them the full extent of the prolapse and my bathroom habits. They just learned to wait for me.

I told none of my women friends until I decided to have surgery. I did not want anyone picturing the bulge between my legs when they looked at me.

Until age 62, I had always been a very sexual woman. I had stopped meeting men at that point since my romantic life had all too often been a disappointment. I was happier doing arts and crafts, working on the family business, watching shows and reading. I recently read a great comment from a woman on Facebook who said, *"Romance doesn't make you happy. New art supplies do!"* I agreed!

When Dr. Chiodi told me I would not be able to have intercourse ever again after the surgery I said it was fine with me. I just wanted to feel comfortable and normal. In this text I have mentioned several times the result of the surgery in order to make sure no one misses the point. You will be making an irreversible choice. Many doctors who perform Colpocleisis surgery will not agree to do it on a woman under the age of 80.

Internal pessaries are prescribed by doctors to brace a first or second degree prolapse. They must be fitted. A pessary will simply fall out if placed in the vagina of a woman with 3-4 degree prolapse. The prolapse muscle is so strong it just pushes it out the minute she stands up. Pessaries also have their own set of complications. You can look up information on them online.

After 6 months with complete prolapse I found a pelvic prolapse brace on the internet. It was tight and uncomfortable but it kept the prolapse supported about 50% - 75% of the way. It allowed me to walk around feeling less vulnerable, however the idea of wearing it for the rest of my life was depressing. I was also worried that if I became old and infirm, I would not be able to empty my bladder if I couldn't remember to splint. It was a scary thought.

Now that the surgery has been a total success, I decided to find other uses for the pelvic belts. After all, 2 belts cost me over $100. I cut out the crotch parts and kept the rest since it is a very strong Velcro material. I have found excellent uses for the Velcro. I lean toward the practical.

Had I known about Le Fort Colpocleisis Surgery when I first experienced the complete prolapse, I would have opted for it immediately. Knowledge of this surgery is too uncommon and doctors too often neglect to mention it as an option. This is one of the reasons I've written this book.

The Last GYN Exam Ever!

Over the next five weeks I experienced the stitches dropping out, but first they would start to unravel as little curly bits. They would stick into my skin like little barbs. With the permission of the doctor's nurse, I used Aquaphor Healing Ointment which helped. The stitches would unravel a little more and eventually drop down and out. This fun sequence went on until six weeks and two days after the surgery when magically they were all gone! Happy Day!

Six weeks after surgery I had my check up with Dr. Chiodi. As usual she was smiling, friendly and welcoming. She checked my new upholstery and declared it healed perfectly. She said I would not be seeing her again. I told her about this book and received permission to mention her in it. I told her I would send her a copy. She replied that she will be excited to get it.

I had sent her a pre-surgery shopping list for her patients. It was the same information I have supplied from pages 22-25. She said she had been giving it to patients and they found it helpful. I was very glad to have been of some service to women facing this difficult time.

When the healing was complete, I looked with a mirror and found it looked the same from the outside as it did before the prolapse. I touched the area and sure enough it was about one inch deep and 1 inch wide. Even though I knew intellectually that this is what I would find it was still a shock. The reality sunk in and for a few hours I felt down. Then remembering how lucky I was not to have this horrible bulge anymore I felt better.

My goal with this book is to help you get through this situation by feeling like you have a sister by your side. It is my hope that his book helps you decide what is best for you by explaining in detail what I experienced.

My email is:

JudithCutlerBook@gmail.com

if you wish to write to me with questions, notes or comments I would love to hear from you. I will always answer. Thank you for buying my book and I hope it helps make your life better.

My blog is:
vaginalprolapse.blogspot.com

www.ingramcontent.com/pod-product-compliance
Lightning Source LLC
Chambersburg PA
CBHW062104270326
41931CB00013B/3211